The Definitive Keto Vegetarian Cooking Guide

Don't Miss Out These Healthy and Delicious Recipes for Busy People

Tia Graham

Table of contents

3

Grilled Portobello with Mashed Potatoes and Green Beans

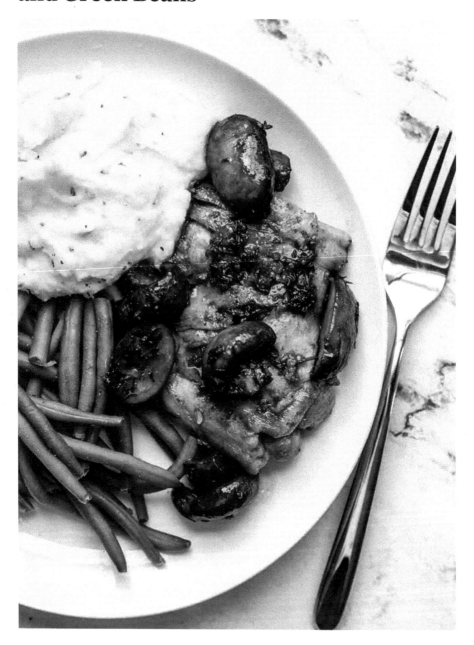

Preparation time: 20 minutes cooking time: 40 minutes servings: 4

Ingredients

For the grilled portobellos

4 large portobello mushrooms

1 teaspoon olive oil

Pinch sea salt

For the mashed potatoes

6 large potatoes, scrubbed or peeled, and chopped

3 to 4 garlic cloves, minced

½ teaspoon olive oil

½ cup non-dairy milk

2 tablespoons coconut oil (optional

2 tablespoons nutritional yeast (optional Pinch sea salt)

For the green beans

2 cups green beans, cut into 1-inch pieces

2 to 3 teaspoons coconut oil

Pinch sea salt

1 to 2 tablespoons nutritional yeast (optional

Directions

To Make The Grilled Portobellos

1.   Preheat the grill to medium, or the oven to 350°F.

2.   Take the stems out of the mushrooms.

3.   Wipe the caps clean with a damp paper towel, then dry them. Spray the caps with a bit of olive oil, or put some oil in your hand and rub it over the mushrooms.

4.   Rub the oil onto the top and bottom of each mushroom, then sprinkle them with a bit of salt on top and bottom.

5.   Put them bottom side facing up on a baking sheet in the oven, or straight on the grill. They'll take about 30 minutes in the oven, or 20 minutes on the grill. Wait until they're soft and wrinkling around the edges. If you keep them bottom up, all the delicious mushroom juice will pool in the cap. Then at the very end, you can flip them over to drain the juice. If you like it, you can drizzle it over the mashed potatoes.

To Make The Mashed Potatoes

6.   Boil the chopped potatoes in lightly salted water for about 20 minutes, until soft. While they're cooking, sauté the garlic in the olive oil, or bake them whole in a 350°F oven for 10 minutes, then squeeze out the flesh. Drain the potatoes, reserving about ½ cup water to mash them. In a large bowl, mash the potatoes with a little bit of the reserved water, the cooked garlic, milk, coconut oil (if using), nutritional yeast (if using), and salt to taste. Add more water, a little at a time, if needed, to get the texture you want. If you use an immersion blender or beater to purée them, you'll have some extra-creamy potatoes.

To Make The Green Bean

7.   Heat a medium pot with a small amount of water to boil, then steam the green beans by either putting them directly in the pot or in a steaming basket.

8.   Once they're slightly soft and vibrantly green, 7 to 8 minutes, take them off the heat and toss them with

the oil, salt, and nutritional yeast (if using).

Nutrition: Calories: 263; Total fat: 7g; Carbs: 43g; Fiber: 7g; Protein: 10g

Tahini Broccoli Slaw

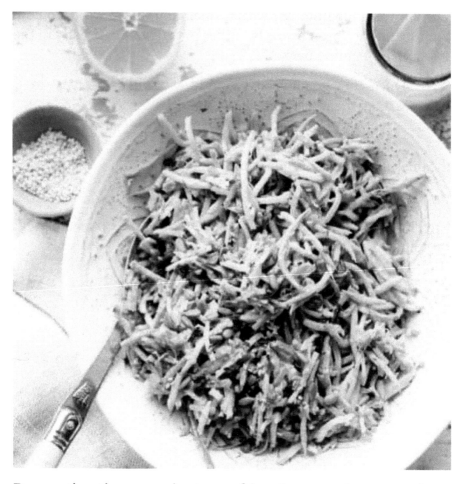

Preparation time: 15 minutes cooking time: 0 minutes servings: 4 to 6

Ingredients

¼ cup tahini (sesame paste 2 tablespoons white miso)

1 tablespoon rice vinegar

1 tablespoon toasted sesame oil

2 teaspoons soy sauce

1 (12-ouncebag broccoli slaw

2 green onions, minced

¼ cup toasted sesame seeds

Directions

1.　　In a large bowl, whisk together the tahini, miso, vinegar, oil, and soy sauce. Add the broccoli slaw, green onions, and sesame seeds and toss to coat.

2.　　Set aside for 20 minutes before serving.

Steamed Cauliflower

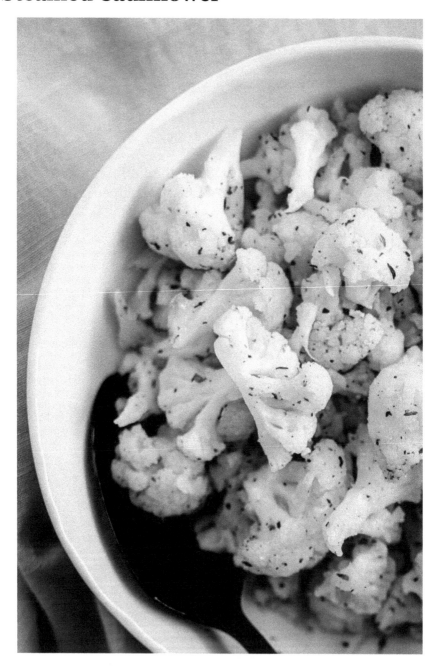

Preparation time: 5 minutes cooking time: 10 minutes servings: 6

Ingredients

1 large head cauliflower 1

 cup water

½ teaspoon salt

1 teaspoon red pepper flakes (optional

Directions

1.   Remove any leaves from the cauliflower, and cut it into florets.

2.   In a large saucepan, bring the water to a boil. Place a steamer basket over the water, and add the florets and salt. Cover and steam for 5 to 7 minutes, until tender. In a large bowl, toss the cauliflower with the red pepper flakes (if using). Transfer the florets to a large airtight container or 6 single-serving containers. Let cool before sealing the lids.

Nutrition: Calories: 35; Fat: 0g; Protein: 3g; Carbohydrates: 7g; Fiber: 4g; Sugar: 4g; Sodium: 236mg

Roasted Cauliflower Tacos

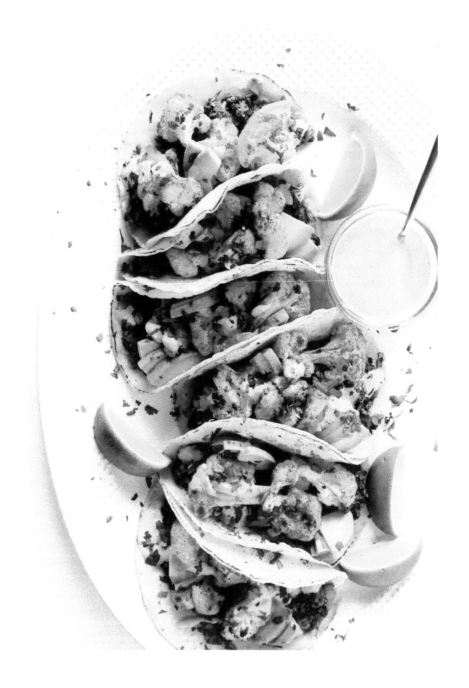

Preparation time: 10 minutes cooking time: 30 minutes Servings: 8 TACOS

Ingredients

For the roasted cauliflower

1   head cauliflower, cut into bite-size pieces

1 tablespoon olive oil (optional

2   tablespoons whole-wheat flour

2 tablespoons nutritional yeast

For the tacos

1   to 2 teaspoons smoked paprika

½ to 1 teaspoon chili powder Pinch sea salt

2   cups shredded lettuce

2 cups cherry tomatoes, quartered

2 carrots, scrubbed or peeled, and grated

½ cup Fresh Mango Salsa

½ cup Guacamole

8 small whole-grain or corn tortillas

1 lime, cut into 8 wedges

Directions

To Make The Roasted Cauliflower

1.   Preheat the oven to 350°F. Lightly grease a large rectangular baking sheet with olive oil, or line it with parchment paper. In a large bowl, toss the cauliflower pieces with oil (if using), or just rinse them so they're wet. The idea is to get the seasonings to stick. In a smaller bowl, mix together the flour, nutritional yeast, paprika, chili powder, and salt.

2.   Add the seasonings to the cauliflower, and mix it around with your hands to thoroughly coat. Spread the cauliflower on the baking sheet, and roast for 20 to 30 minutes, or until softened.

To Make The Tacos.

3.   Prep the veggies, salsa, and guacamole while the cauliflower is roasting. Once the cauliflower is cooked, heat the tortillas for just a few minutes in the oven or in a small skillet. Set everything out on the table, and assemble your tacos as you go. Give a squeeze of fresh lime just before eating.

Nutrition (1 taco): Calories: 198; Total fat: 6g; Carbs: 32g; Fiber: 6g; Protein: 7g

Cajun Sweet

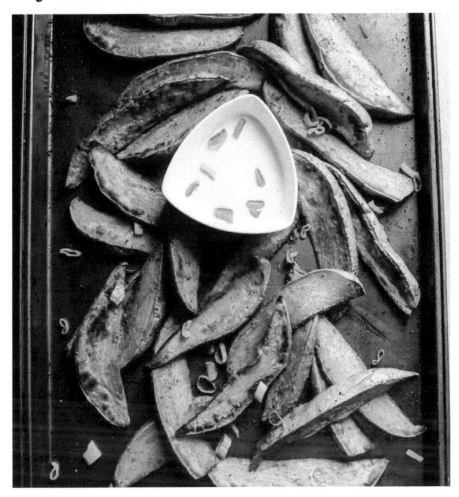

Potatoes Preparation time: 5 minutes cooking time: 30 minutes servings: 4

Ingredients

2 pounds sweet potatoes

2 teaspoons extra-virgin olive oil

½ teaspoon ground cayenne pepper

½ teaspoon smoked paprika

½ teaspoon dried oregano

½ teaspoon dried thyme

½ teaspoon garlic powder

½ teaspoon salt (optional

Directions

1.	Preheat the oven to 400°F. Line a baking sheet with parchment paper.

2.	Wash the potatoes, pat dry, and cut into ¾-inch cubes. Transfer to a large bowl, and pour the olive oil over the potatoes.

3.	In a small bowl, combine the cayenne, paprika, oregano, thyme, and garlic powder. Sprinkle the spices over the potatoes and combine until the potatoes are well coated. Spread the potatoes on the prepared baking sheet in a single layer. Season with the salt (if using). Roast for 30 minutes, stirring the potatoes after 15 minutes.

4.	Divide the potatoes evenly among 4 single-serving containers. Let cool completely before sealing.

Nutrition: Calories: 219; Fat: 3g; Protein: 4g; Carbohydrates: 46g; Fiber: 7g; Sugar: 9g; Sodium: 125mg

Creamy Mint-Lime Spaghetti Squash

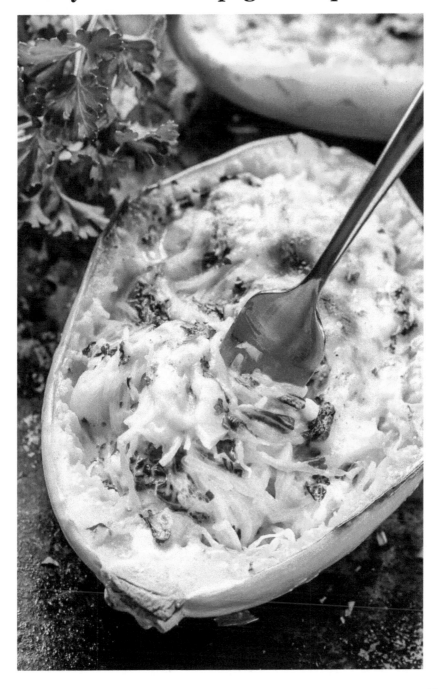

Preparation time: 10 minutes cooking time: 30 minutes servings: 3

Ingredients

For the dressing

3 tablespoons tahini

Zest and juice of 1 small lime

2 tablespoons fresh mint, minced

1 small garlic clove, pressed

1 tablespoon nutritional yeast Pinch sea salt

For the spaghetti squash

1 spaghetti squash

Pinch sea salt

1 cup cherry tomatoes, chopped

1 cup chopped bell pepper, any color

Freshly ground black pepper

Directions

To Make The Dressing

1.   Make the dressing by whisking together the tahini and lime juice until thick, stirring in water if you need it, until smooth,

then add the rest of the ingredients. Or you can purée all the ingredients in a blender.

To Make The Spaghetti Squash.

2.	Put a large pot of water on high and bring to a boil. Cut the squash in half and scoop out the seeds. Put the squash halves in the pot with the salt, and boil for about 30 minutes. Carefully remove the squash from the pot and let it cool until you can safely handle it. Set half the squash aside for another meal. Scoop out the squash from the skin, which stays hard like a shell, and break the strands apart. The flesh absorbs water while boiling, so set the "noodles" in a strainer for 10 minutes, tossing occasionally to drain. Transfer the cooked spaghetti squash to a large bowl and toss with the mint-lime dressing. Then top with the cherry tomatoes and bell pepper. Add an extra sprinkle of nutritional yeast and black pepper, if you wish.

Nutrition: Calories: 199; Total fat: 10g; Carbs: 27g; Fiber: 5g;

Smoky Coleslaw

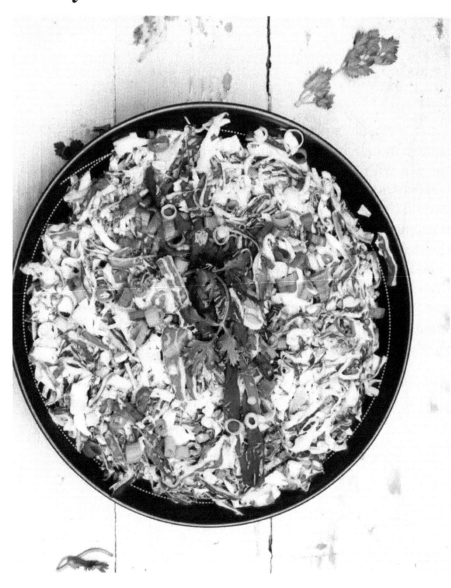

Preparation time: 10 minutes cooking time: 0 minutes servings: 6

Ingredients

1 pound shredded cabbage

⅓ cup vegan mayonnaise

¼ cup unseasoned rice vinegar

3 tablespoons plain vegan yogurt or plain soymilk

1 tablespoon vegan sugar

½ teaspoon salt

¼ teaspoon freshly ground black pepper

¼ teaspoon smoked paprika

¼ teaspoon chipotle powder

Directions

1.   Put the shredded cabbage in a large bowl. In a medium bowl, whisk the mayonnaise, vinegar, yogurt, sugar, salt, pepper, paprika, and chipotle powder.

2.   Pour over the cabbage, and mix with a spoon or spatula and until the cabbage shreds are coated. Divide the coleslaw evenly among 6 single-serving containers. Seal the lids.

Nutrition: Calories: 73; Fat: 4g; Protein: 1g; Carbohydrates: 8g; Fiber: 2g; Sugar: 5g; Sodium: 283mg

Simple Sesame Stir-Fry

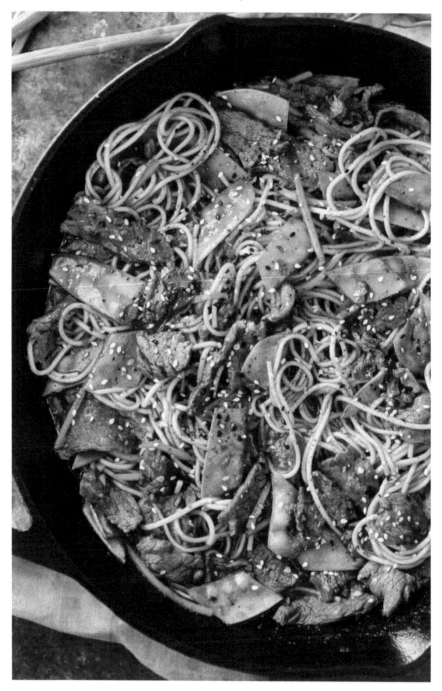

Preparation time: 10 minutes cooking time: 20 minutes

servings: 4

Ingredients

1   cup quinoa

2   cups water Pinch sea salt

1 head broccoli

1 to 2 teaspoons untoasted sesame oil, or olive oil

1   cup snow peas, or snap peas, ends trimmed and cut in half

1 cup frozen shelled edamame beans, or peas

2   cups chopped Swiss chard, or other large-leafed green

2 scallions, chopped

2 tablespoons water

1 teaspoon toasted sesame oil

1 tablespoon tamari, or soy sauce

2 tablespoons sesame seeds

Directions

1.   Put the quinoa, water, and sea salt in a medium pot, bring it to a boil for a minute, then turn to low and simmer, covered, for 20 minutes. The quinoa is fully cooked when you see the swirl of the grains with a translucent center, and it is fluffy. Do not stir the quinoa while it is cooking.

2.   Meanwhile, cut the broccoli into bite-size florets, cutting and pulling apart from the stem. Also chop the stem into bite-size

pieces. Heat a large skillet to high, and sauté the broccoli in the untoasted sesame oil, with a pinch of salt to help it soften. Keep this moving continuously, so that it doesn't burn, and add an extra drizzle of oil if needed as you add the rest of the vegetables. Add the snow peas next, continuing to stir. Add the edamame until they thaw. Add the Swiss chard and scallions at the same time, tossing for only a minute to wilt. Then add 2 tablespoons of water to the hot skillet so that it sizzles and finishes the vegetables with a quick steam.

3.   Dress with the toasted sesame oil and tamari, and toss one last time. Remove from the heat immediately. Serve a scoop of cooked quinoa, topped with stir-fry and sprinkled with some sesame seeds, and an extra drizzle of tamari and/or toasted sesame oil if you like.

Nutrition: Calories: 334; Total fat: 13g; Carbs: 42g; Fiber: 9g; Protein: 17g

Mediterranean Hummus Pizza

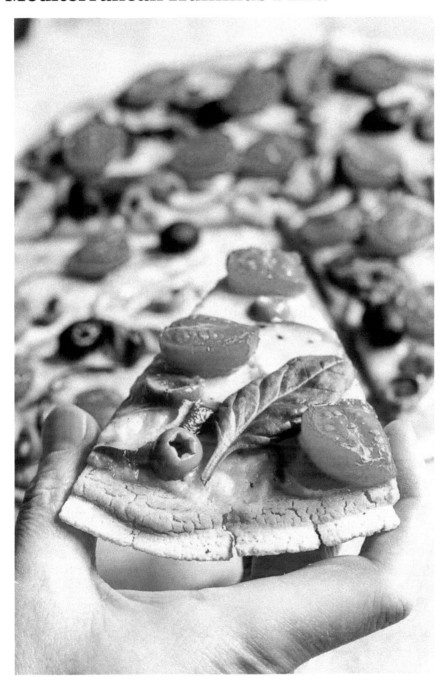

Preparation time: 10 minutes cooking time: 30 minutes servings: 2 pizzas

Ingredients

½ zucchini, thinly sliced

½ red onion, thinly sliced

1   cup cherry tomatoes, halved

2   to 4 tablespoons pitted and chopped black olives

Pinch sea salt

Drizzle olive oil (optional 2 prebaked pizza crusts

½ cup Classic Hummus, or Roasted Red Pepper Hummus

2 to 4 tablespoons Cheesy Sprinkle

Directions

1.   Preheat the oven to 400°F. Place the zucchini, onion, cherry tomatoes, and olives in a large bowl, sprinkle them with the sea salt, and toss them a bit. Drizzle with a bit of olive oil (if using), to seal in the flavor and keep them from drying out in the oven.

2.   Lay the two crusts out on a large baking sheet. Spread half the hummus on each crust, and top with the veggie mixture and some Cheesy Sprinkle. Pop the pizzas in the oven for 20 to 30 minutes, or until the veggies are soft.

Nutrition (1 pizzaCalories: 500; Total fat: 25g; Carbs: 58g; Fiber: 12g; Protein: 19g

Baked Brussels Sprouts

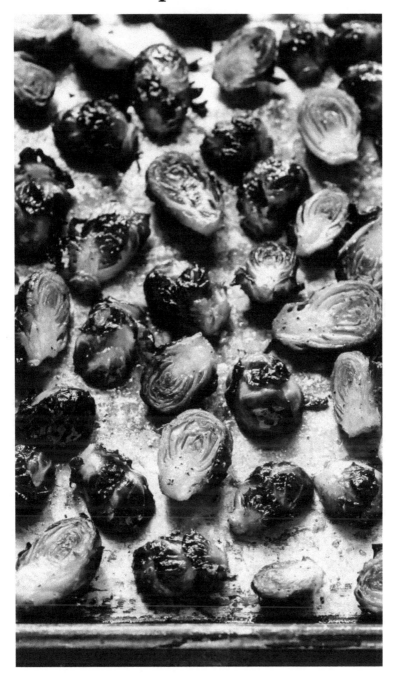

Preparation time: 10 minutes cooking time: 40 minutes servings: 4

Ingredients

1   pound Brussels sprouts

2   teaspoons extra-virgin olive or canola oil

4 teaspoons minced garlic (about 4 cloves 1 teaspoon dried oregano

½ teaspoon dried rosemary

½ teaspoon salt

¼ teaspoon freshly ground black pepper

1 tablespoon balsamic vinegar

Directions

1.   Preheat the oven to 400°F. Line a rimmed baking sheet with parchment paper. Trim and halve the Brussels sprouts. Transfer to a large bowl. Toss with the olive oil, garlic, oregano, rosemary, salt, and pepper to coat well.

2.   Transfer to the prepared baking sheet. Bake for 35 to 40 minutes, shaking the pan occasionally to help with even browning, until crisp on the outside and tender on the inside. Remove from the oven and transfer to a large bowl. Stir in the balsamic vinegar, coating well.

3.   Divide the Brussels sprouts evenly among 4 single-serving containers. Let cool before sealing the lids.

Nutrition: Calories: 77; Fat: 3g; Protein: 4g; Carbohydrates: 12g; Fiber: 5g; Sugar: 3g; Sodium: 320mg

Minted Peas

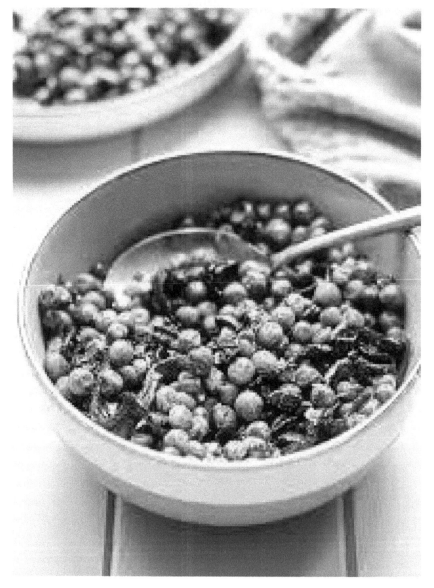

Preparation time: 5 minutes cooking time: 5 minutes servings: 4

Ingredients

1 tablespoon olive oil

4 cups peas, fresh or frozen (not canned

½ teaspoon sea salt

freshly ground black pepper

3 tablespoons chopped fresh mint

Directions

1.   In a large sauté pan, heat the olive oil over medium-high heat until hot. Add the peas and cook, about 5 minutes.

2.   Remove the pan from heat. Stir in the salt, season with pepper, and stir in the mint.

3.   Serve hot.

Edamame Donburi

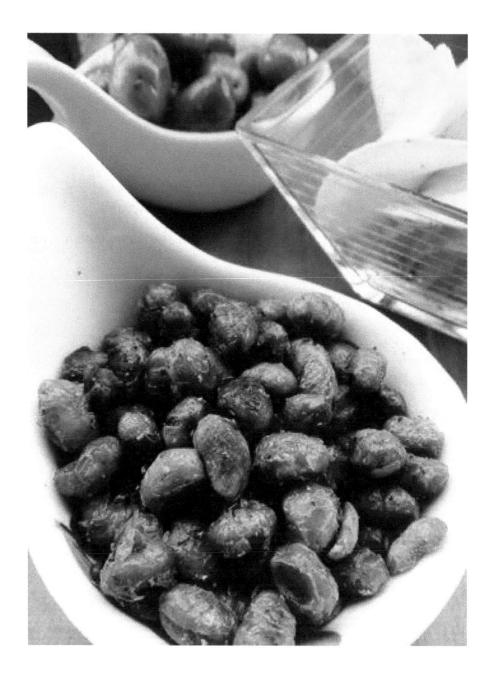

Preparation time: 5 minutes cooking time: 20 minutes servings: 4

Ingredients

1 cup fresh or frozen shelled edamame

1 tablespoon canola or grapeseed oil

1 medium yellow onion, minced

5 shiitake mushroom caps, lightly rinsed, patted dry, and cut into 1/4-inch strips

1 teaspoon grated fresh ginger

3 green onions, minced

8 ounces firm tofu, drained and crumbled

2 tablespoons soy sauce

3 cups hot cooked white or brown rice

1 tablespoon toasted sesame oil

1   tablespoon toasted sesame seeds, for garnish

Directions

1.   In a small saucepan of boiling salted water, cook the edamame until tender, about 10 minutes. Drain and set aside.

2.   In a large skillet, heat the canola oil over medium heat. Add the onion, cover, and cook until softened, about 5 minutes. Add the mushrooms and cook, uncovered, 5 minutes longer. Stir in the ginger and green onions. Add the tofu and soy sauce and cook until heated through, stirring to combine well, about 5 minutes.

Stir in the cooked edamame and cook until heated through, about 5 minutes.

3.   Divide the hot rice among 4 bowls, top each with the edamame and tofu mixture, and drizzle on the sesame oil. Sprinkle with sesame seeds and serve immediately.

Sicilian Stuffed Tomatoes

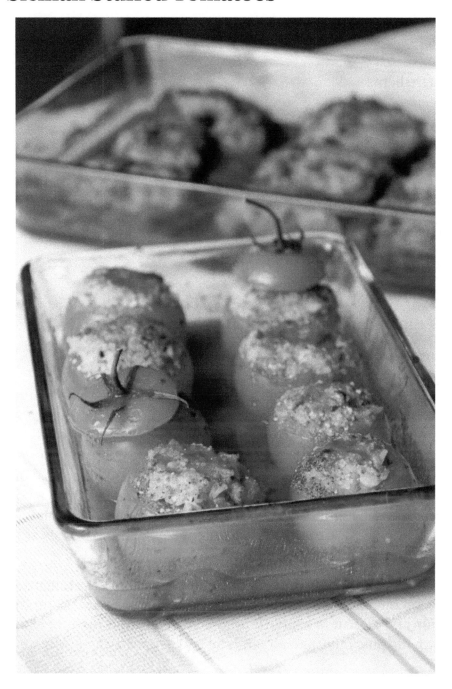

Preparation time: 10 minutes cooking time: 30 minutes

servings: 4

Ingredients

2   cups water

1 cup couscous Salt

3 green onions, minced

1/3 cup golden raisins

1 teaspoon finely grated orange zest

4 large ripe tomatoes

1/3 cup toasted pine nuts

1/4 cup minced fresh parsley

Freshly ground black pepper

2 teaspoons olive oil

Directions

1.   Preheat the oven to 375°F. Lightly oil a 9 x 13-inch baking pan and set aside. In a large saucepan, bring the water to a boil over high heat. Stir in the couscous and salt to taste and remove from the heat. Stir in the green onions, raisins, and orange zest. Cover and set aside for 5 minutes.

2.   Cut a 1/2-inch-thick slice off the top of each of the tomatoes. Scoop out the pulp, keeping the tomato shells intact. Chop the pulp and place it in a large bowl. Add the couscous mixture along with the pine nuts, parsley, and salt and pepper to taste. Mix well.

3.   Fill the tomatoes with the mixture and place them in the prepared pan. Drizzle the tomatoes with the oil, cover with foil, and bake until hot, about 20 minutes. Serve immediately.

Basic Baked

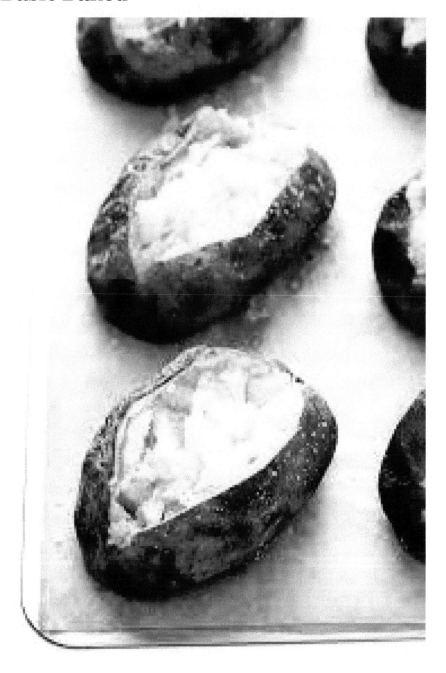

Potatoes Preparation time: 5 minutes cooking time: 60 minutes servings: 5

Ingredients

1.   5 medium Russet potatoes or a variety of potatoes, washed and patted dry

2.   1 to 2 tablespoons extra-virgin olive oil or aquafaba (see tip

3.   ¼ teaspoon salt

4.   ¼ teaspoon freshly ground black pepper

Directions

1.   Preheat the oven to 400°F. Pierce each potato several times with a fork or a knife. Brush the olive oil over the potatoes, then rub each with a pinch of the salt and a pinch of the pepper.

2.   Place the potatoes on a baking sheet and bake for 50 to 60 minutes, until tender. Place the potatoes on a baking rack and cool completely. Transfer to an airtight container or 5 single-serving containers. Let cool before sealing the lids.

Nutrition: Calories: 171; Fat: 3g; Protein: 4g; Carbohydrates: 34g; Fiber: 5g; Sugar: 3g; Sodium: 129mg

Orange-Dressed Asparagus

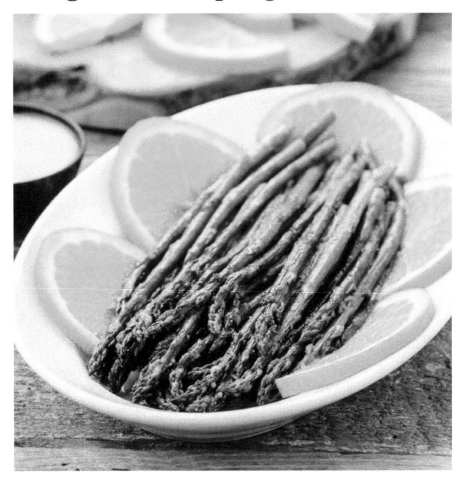

Preparation time: 5 minutes cooking time: 10 minutes servings: 4

Ingredients

1 medium shallot, minced

2 teaspoons orange zest

1/3 cup fresh orange juice

1   tablespoon fresh lemon juice Pinch sugar

2   tablespoons olive oil

Salt and freshly ground black pepper

1 pound asparagus, tough ends trimmed

Directions

1.   In a small bowl, combine the shallot, orange zest, orange juice, lemon juice, sugar, and oil. Add salt and pepper to taste and mix well. Set aside to allow flavors to blend, for 5 to 10 minutes.

2.   Steam the asparagus until just tender, 4 to 5 minutes. If serving hot, arrange on a serving platter and drizzle the dressing over the asparagus. Serve at once.

3.   If serving chilled, run the asparagus under cold water to stop the cooking process and retain the color. Drain on paper towels, then cover and refrigerate until chilled, about 1 hour. To serve, arrange the asparagus on a serving platter and drizzle with the dressing.

Broccoli With Almonds

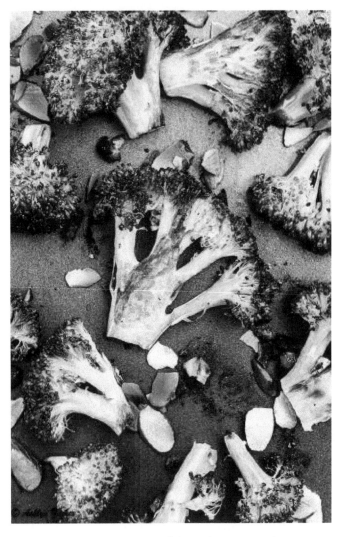

Preparation time: 5 minutes cooking time: 15 minutes servings: 4

Ingredients

1 pound broccoli, cut into small florets

2 tablespoons olive oil

3 garlic cloves, minced

1   cup thinly sliced white mushrooms

1/4 cup dry white wine

2   tablespoons minced fresh parsley

Salt and freshly ground black pepper

1/2 cup slivered toasted almonds

Directions

1.   Steam the broccoli until just tender, about 5 minutes. Run under cold water and set aside.

2.   In a large skillet, heat 1 tablespoon of the oil over medium heat. Add the garlic and mushrooms and cook until soft, about 5 minutes. Add the wine and cook 1 minute longer. Add the steamed broccoli and parsley and season with salt and pepper to taste. Cook until the liquid is evaporated and the broccoli is hot, about 3 minutes.

3.   Transfer to a serving bowl, drizzle with the remaining 1 tablespoon oil and the almonds, and toss to coat. Serve immediately.

Glazed Curried Carrots

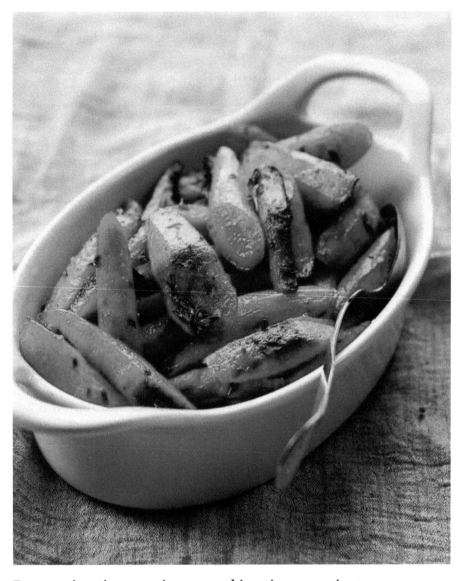

Preparation time: 5 minutes cooking time: 15 minutes

servings: 6

Ingredients

1   pound carrots, peeled and thinly sliced 2 tablespoons olive oil

2   tablespoons curry powder

2 tablespoons pure maple syrup juice of ½ lemon

sea salt

freshly ground black pepper

Directions

1.   Place the carrots in a large pot and cover with water. Cook on medium-high heat until tender, about 10 minutes. Drain the carrots and return them to the pan over medium-low heat.

2.   Stir in the olive oil, curry powder, maple syrup, and lemon juice. Cook, stirring constantly, until the liquid reduces, about 5 minutes. Season with salt and pepper and serve immediately.

Miso Spaghetti Squash

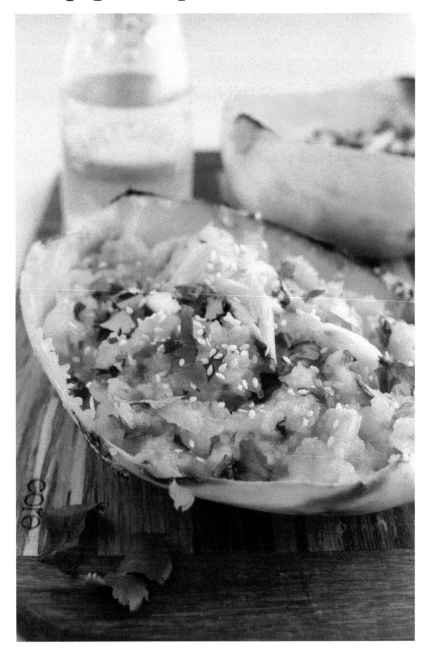

Preparation time: 5 minutes cooking time: 40 minutes servings: 4

Ingredients

1 (3-poundspaghetti squash

1 tablespoon hot water

1   tablespoon unseasoned rice vinegar

1 tablespoon white miso

Directions

1.   Preheat the oven to 400°F. Line a rimmed baking sheet with parchment paper. Halve the squash lengthwise and place, cut-side down, on the prepared baking sheet.

2.   Bake for 35 to 40 minutes, until tender. Cool until the squash is easy to handle. With a fork, scrape out the flesh, which will be stringy, like spaghetti. Transfer to a large bowl. In a small bowl, combine the hot water, vinegar, and miso with a whisk or fork. Pour over the squash. Gently toss with tongs to coat the squash. Divide the squash evenly among 4 single-serving containers. Let cool before sealing the lids.

Nutrition: Calories: 117; Fat: 2g; Protein: 3g; Carbohydrates: 25g; Fiber: 0g; Sugar: 0g; Sodium: 218mg

Braised Cabbage And Apples

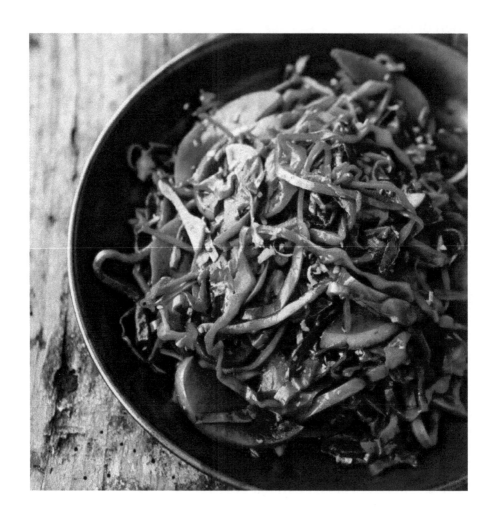

Preparation time: 5 minutes cooking time: 25 minutes servings: 6

Ingredients

2   tablespoons olive oil

1 small head red cabbage, shredded

1 small head savoy cabbage, shredded

1 Granny Smith apple

1 red cooking apple, such as Rome or Gala

2 tablespoons sugar

1   cup water

1/4 cup cider vinegar

Salt and freshly ground black pepper

Directions

1.   In a large saucepan, heat the oil over medium heat. Add the shredded red and savoy cabbage, cover, and cook until slightly wilted, 5 minutes.

2.   Core the apples and cut them into 1/4-inch dice. Add the apples to the cabbage, along with the sugar, water, vinegar, and salt and pepper to taste. Reduce heat to low, cover, and simmer until the cabbage and apples are tender, stirring frequently, about 20 minutes. Serve immediately.

Marsala Carrots

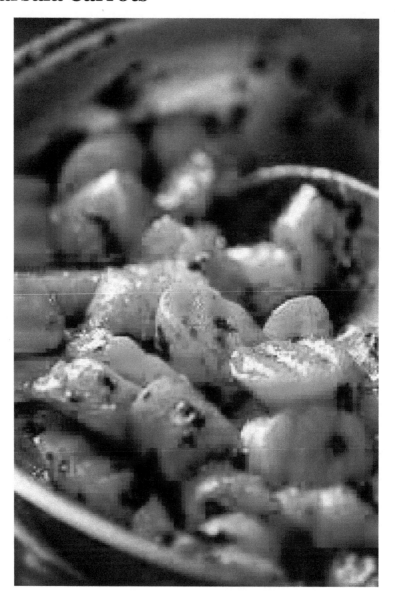

Preparation time: 5 minutes cooking time: 20 minutes servings: 4

Ingredients

2   tablespoons vegan margarine

1 pound carrots, cut diagonally into 1/4-inch slices

Salt and freshly ground black pepper

1/2 cup Marsala

1/4 cup water

1/4 cup chopped fresh parsley, for garnish

Directions

1.   In a large skillet, melt the margarine over medium heat. Add the carrots and toss well to coat evenly with the margarine. Cover and cook, stirring occasionally, for 5 minutes.

2.   Season with salt and pepper to taste, tossing to coat. Add the Marsala and water. Reduce heat to low, cover, and simmer until the carrots are tender, about 15 minutes.

3.   Uncover and cook over medium-high heat until the liquid is reduced into a syrupy sauce, stirring to prevent burning.

4.   Transfer to a serving bowl and sprinkle with parsley. Serve immediately.

Garlic And Herb Zoodles

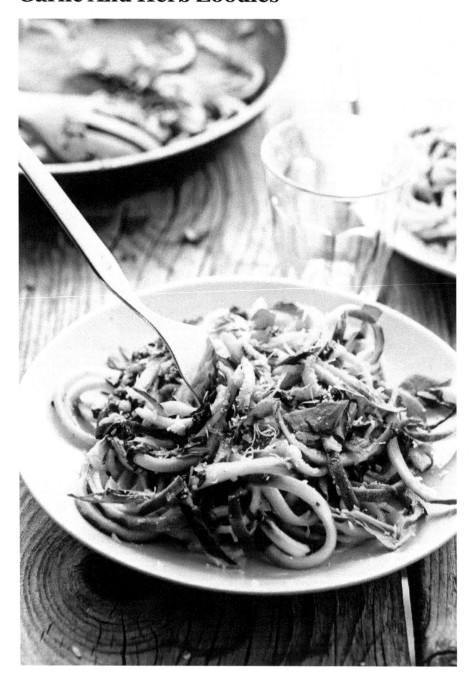

Preparation time: 10 minutes cooking time: 2 minutes

servings: 4

Ingredients

1 teaspoon extra-virgin olive oil or 2 tablespoons vegetable broth

1 teaspoon minced garlic (about 1 clove

4 medium zucchini, spiralized

½ teaspoon dried basil

½ teaspoon dried oregano

¼ to ½ teaspoon red pepper flakes, to taste

¼ teaspoon salt (optional

¼ teaspoon freshly ground black pepper

Directions

1.   In a large skillet over medium-high heat, heat the olive oil.

2.   Add the garlic, zucchini, basil, oregano, red pepper flakes, salt (if using), and black pepper. Sauté for 1 to 2 minutes, until barely tender. Divide the zoodles evenly among 4 storage containers. Let cool before sealing the lids.

Nutrition: Calories: 44; Fat: 2g; Protein: 3g; Carbohydrates: 7g; Fiber: 2g; Sugar: 3g; Sodium: 20mg

Ratatouille (Pressure cooker)

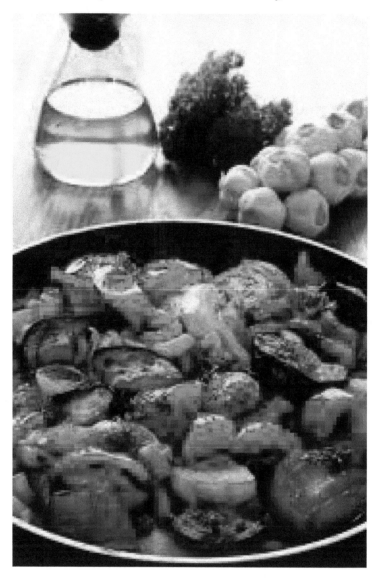

Preparation time: 15 minutes Servings: 4-6

Ingredients

1 onion, diced

4 garlic cloves, minced

1 to 2 teaspoons olive oil

1 cup water

3 or 4 tomatoes, diced

1 eggplant, cubed

1 or 2 bell peppers, any color, seeded and chopped

1½ tablespoons dried herbes de Provence (or any mixture of dried basil, oregano, thyme, marjoram, and rosemary

½ teaspoon salt

Freshly ground black pepper

Directions

1.   On your electric pressure cooker, select Sauté. Add the onion, garlic, and olive oil. Cook for 4 to 5 minutes, stirring occasionally, until the onion is softened. Add the water, tomatoes, eggplant, bell peppers, and herbes de Provence. Cancel Sauté.

2.   High pressure for 6 minutes. Close and lock the lid and ensure the pressure valve is sealed, then select High Pressure and set the time for 6 minutes.

3.   Pressure Release. Once the cook time is complete, let the pressure release naturally, about 20 minutes. Once all the

pressure has released, carefully unlock and remove the lid. Let cool for a few minutes, then season with salt and pepper.

Nutrition Calories: 101; Total fat: 2g; Protein: 4g; Sodium: 304mg; Fiber: 7g

Cardamom Carrots With Orange

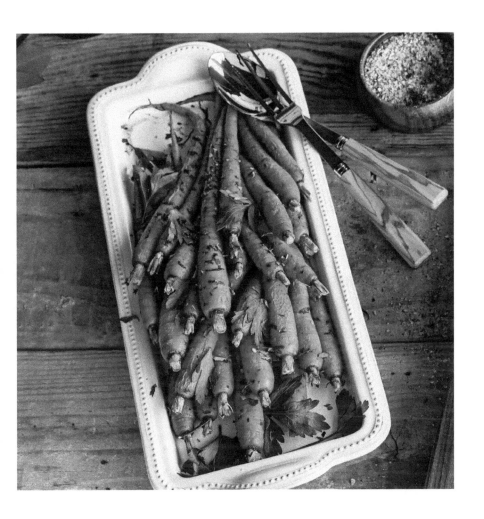

Preparation time: 5 minutes cooking time: 10 minutes

servings: 4

Ingredients

1 pound carrots, cut into 1/4-inch slices

2 tablespoons vegan margarine

1 tablespoon finely grated orange zest

1/2 teaspoon ground cardamom

Salt

Ground cayenne

Directions

1.   Steam the carrots until tender, about 7 minutes. Set aside.

2.   In a large skillet, melt the margarine over medium heat. Add the carrots, orange zest, and cardamom and season with salt and cayenne to taste. Cook, stirring occasionally, until flavors are blended, about 2 minutes. Serve immediately

Stuffed Baby Peppers

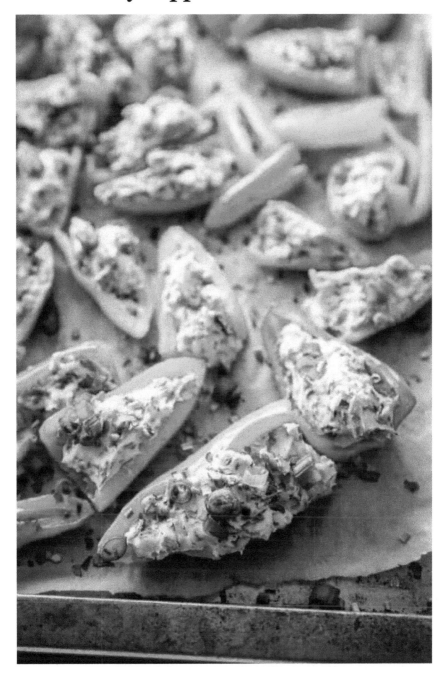

Preparation time: 10 minutes Cooking time: 0 minutes Servings: 4

Ingredients:

12 baby bell peppers, cut into halves lengthwise and seeds removed

¼ teaspoon red pepper flakes, crushed

1 pound shrimp, cooked, peeled and deveined

6 tablespoons jarred Paleo pesto

A pinch of sea salt

Black pepper to taste

1   tablespoon lemon juice

1 tablespoon olive oil

A handful parsley, chopped

Directions:

1.   In a bowl, mix shrimp with pepper flakes, Paleo pesto, a pinch of salt, black pepper, lemon juice, oil and parsley and whisk well.

2.   Divide this into bell pepper halves, arrange on plates and serve.

3.   Enjoy!

Nutritional value/serving: calories 371, fat 14, fiber 3,2, carbs 20,9, protein 30,5

Baked Eggplant

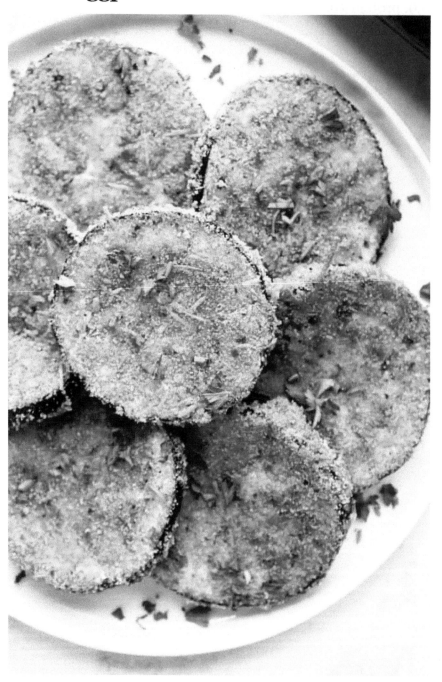

Preparation time: 10 minutes Cooking time: 30 minutes Servings: 3

Ingredients:

2   eggplants, sliced

A pinch of sea salt

Black pepper to taste

1 cup almonds, ground

1 teaspoon garlic, minced

2 teaspoons olive oil

Directions:

1.   Grease a baking dish with some of the oil and arrange eggplant slices on it.

2.   Season them with a pinch of salt and some black pepper and leave them aside for 10 minutes.

3.   In a food processor, mix almonds with the rest of the oil, garlic, a pinch of salt and black pepper and blend well.

4.   Spread this over eggplant slices, place in the oven at 425 degrees F and bake for 30 minutes.

5.   Divide between plates and serve.

6.   Enjoy!

Nutritional value/serving: calories 303, fat 19,6, fiber 16,9, carbs 28,6, protein 10,3

Eggplant Mix

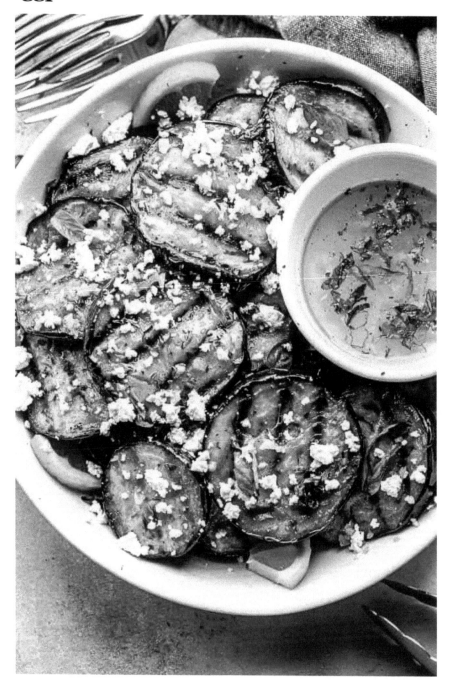

Preparation time: 10 minutes Cooking time: 40 minutes Servings: 3

Ingredients:

5 medium eggplants, sliced into rounds

1 teaspoon thyme, chopped

2 tablespoons balsamic vinegar

1 teaspoon mustard

2 garlic cloves, minced

½ cup olive oil

Black pepper to taste

A pinch of sea salt

1   teaspoon maple syrup

Directions:

1.   In a bowl, mix vinegar with thyme, mustard, garlic, oil, salt, pepper and maple syrup and whisk very well.

2.   Arrange eggplant round on a lined baking sheet, place in the oven at 425 degrees F and roast for 40 minutes.

3.   Divide eggplants between plates and serve.

4.   Enjoy!

Nutritional value/serving: calories 533, fat 35,6, fiber 32,6, carbs 56,5, protein 9,4

Eggplant and Garlic Sauce

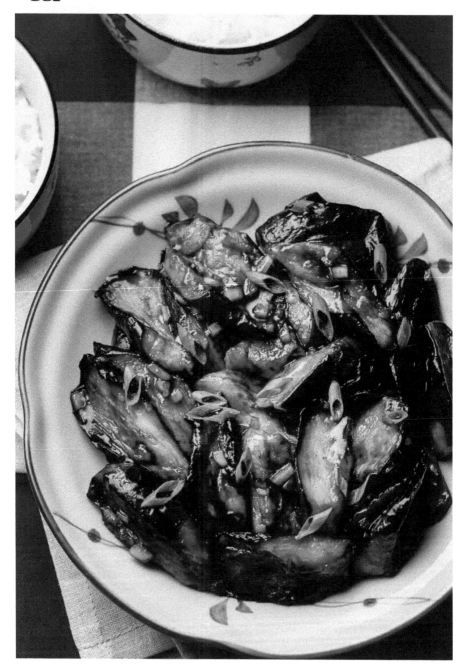

Preparation time: 10 minutes Cooking time: 10 minutes Servings: 4

Ingredients:

2   tablespoons avocado oil

2 garlic cloves, minced

3   eggplants, cut into halves and thinly sliced

1 red chili pepper, chopped

1 green onion stalk, chopped

1 tablespoon ginger, grated

1 tablespoon coconut aminos

1 tablespoon balsamic vinegar

Directions:

1.   Heat up a pan with half of the oil over medium-high heat, add eggplant slices, cook for 2 minutes, flip, cook for 3 minutes more and transfer to a plate.

2.   Heat up the pan with the rest of the oil over medium heat, add chili pepper, garlic, green onions and ginger, stir and cook for 1 minute.

3.   Return eggplant slices to the pan, stir and cook for 1 minute.

4.   Add coconut aminos and vinegar, stir, divide between plates and serve.

5.   Enjoy!

Nutritional value/serving: calories 123, fat 1,7, fiber 15,2, carbs 26,7, protein 4,4

Eggplant Hash

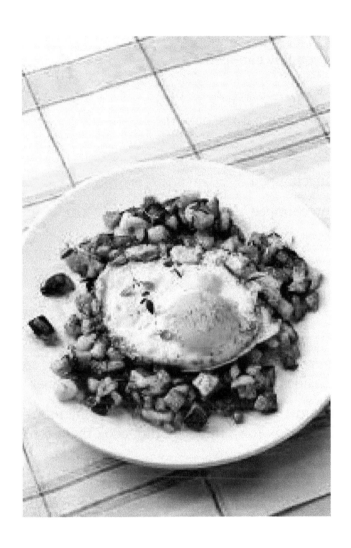

Preparation time: 20 minutes Cooking time: 20 minutes Servings: 4

Ingredients:

1 eggplant, roughly chopped

½ cup olive oil

½ pound cherry tomatoes, halved

1 teaspoon Tabasco sauce

¼ cup basil, chopped

¼ cup mint, chopped

A pinch of sea salt

Black pepper to taste

Directions:

1.   Put eggplant pieces in a bowl, add a pinch of salt, toss to coat, leave aside for 20 minutes and drain using paper towels.

2.   Heat up a pan with half of the oil over medium-high heat, add eggplant, cook for 3 minutes, flip, cook them for 3 minutes more and transfer to a bowl.

3.   Heat up the same pan with the rest of the oil over medium-high heat, add tomatoes and cook them for 8 minutes stirring from time to time.

4.   Return eggplant pieces to the pan and add a pinch of salt, black pepper, basil, mint and Tabasco sauce.

5.   Stir, cook for 2 minutes more, divide between plates and serve.

6. Enjoy!

Nutritional value/serving: calories 258, fat 25,6, fiber 5,1, carbs 9,5, protein 1.9

Eggplant Jam

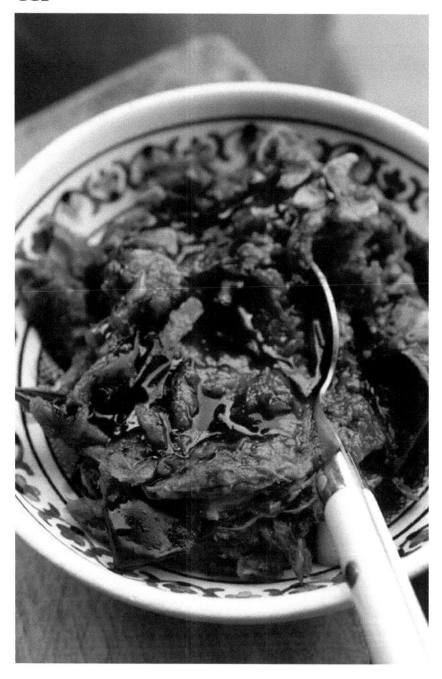

Preparation time: 10 minutes Cooking time: 1 hour Servings: 6

Ingredients:

3 eggplants, sliced lengthwise

2 teaspoons sweet paprika

2 garlic cloves, minced

A pinch of sea salt

A pinch of cinnamon, ground 1teaspoon cumin, ground

A splash of hot sauce

¼ cup water

1 tablespoon parsley, chopped

2 tablespoons lemon juice

Directions:

1.   Sprinkle some salt on eggplant slices and leave them aside for 10 minutes.

2.   Pat dry eggplant, brush them with half of the oil, place on a lined baking sheet, place in the oven at 375

degrees F, bake for 25 minutes flipping them halfway and leave them aside to cool down.

3.   In a bowl, mix paprika with garlic, cinnamon, cumin, water and hot sauce and stir well.

4.   Add baked eggplant pieces and mash them with a fork.

5.   Heat up a pan with the rest of the oil over medium-low heat, add eggplant mix, stir and cook for 20 minutes.

6.   Add lemon juice and parsley, stir, take off heat, divide into small bowls and serve.

7.   Enjoy!

Nutritional value/serving: calories 75, fat 0,7, fiber 10,1, carbs 17,2, protein 3

Warm Watercress Mix

Preparation time: 10 minutes Cooking time: 10 minutes Servings: 4

Ingredients:

1 pound watercress, chopped

¼ cup olive oil

1 garlic clove, cut in halves

1 small shallot, peeled, cooked and chopped

¼ cup hazelnuts, chopped

Black pepper to taste

¼ cup pine nuts

Directions:

1.   Heat up a pan with the oil over medium heat, add garlic clove halves, cook for 2 minutes and discard.

2.   Heat up the pan with the garlic oil again over medium heat, add hazelnuts and pine nuts, stir and cook for 6 minutes.

3.   Add shallots, black pepper to taste and watercress, stir, cook for 2 minutes, divide between plates and serve right away.

4.   Enjoy!

Nutritional value/serving: calories 220, fat 21,8, fiber 2,1, carbs 2,9, protein 5,3

Watercress Soup

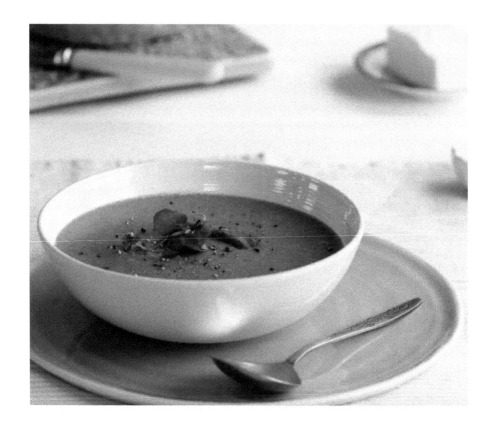

Preparation time: 10 minutes Cooking time: 20 minutes Servings: 4

Ingredients:

8 ounces watercress

1 tablespoon lemon juice

A pinch of nutmeg, ground

4 ounces coconut milk

A pinch of sea salt Black pepper to taste

14 ounces veggie stock

1 celery stick, chopped

1 onion, chopped

1 tablespoon olive oil

12 ounces sweet potatoes, peeled and chopped

Directions:

1.   Heat up a large saucepan with the oil over medium heat, add onion and celery, stir and cook for 5 minutes.

2.   Add sweet potato pieces and stock, stir, bring to a simmer, cover and cook on a low heat for 10 minutes.

3.   Add watercress, stir, cover saucepan again and cook for 5 minutes.

4.   Blend this with an immersion blender, add a pinch of nutmeg, lemon juice, salt, pepper and coconut milk, bring to a simmer again, divide into bowls and serve.

5.   Enjoy!

Nutritional value/serving: calories 224, fat 11,8, fiber 5,7, carbs 29,6, protein 4

Artichokes and Mushroom Mix

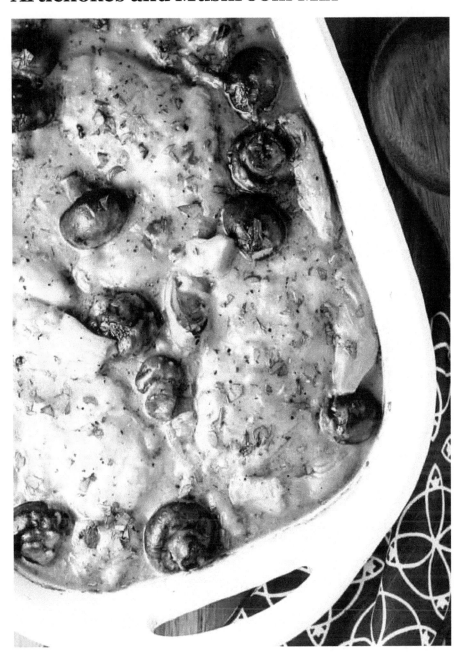

Preparation time: 30 minutes Cooking time: 30 minutes Servings: 4

Ingredients:

16 mushrooms, sliced

1/3 cup tamari sauce

1/3 cup olive oil

4 tablespoons balsamic vinegar

4 garlic cloves, minced

1 tablespoon lemon juice

1 teaspoon oregano, dried

1 teaspoon rosemary, dried

½ tablespoon thyme, dried

A pinch of sea salt

Black pepper to taste

1 sweet onion, chopped

1 jar artichoke hearts

4 cups spinach

1 tablespoon coconut oil

1 teaspoon garlic, minced

1 cauliflower head, florets separated

½ cup veggie stock

1 teaspoon garlic powder

A pinch of nutmeg, ground

Directions:

1.   In a bowl, mix vinegar with tamari sauce, lemon juice, 4 garlic cloves, olive oil, oregano, rosemary, thyme, a pinch of salt, black pepper and mushrooms, toss to coat well and leave aside for 30 minutes.

2.   Transfer these to a lined baking sheet and bake them in the oven at 350 degrees F for 30 minutes.

3.   In a food processor, mix cauliflower with a pinch of sea salt and black pepper and pulse until you obtain rice.

4.   Heat a pan to medium-high heat, add cauliflower rice, toast for 2 minutes, add nutmeg, garlic powder, black pepper and stock, stir and cook until stock evaporated.

5.   Heat a pan with the coconut oil over medium heat, add onion, artichokes, 1 teaspoon garlic and spinach, stir and cook for a few minutes.

6.   Divide cauliflower rice on plates, top with artichokes and mushrooms and serve.

Nutritional value/serving: calories 354, fat 29,9, fiber 4,3, carbs 16,5, protein 6,6

Artichokes with Horseradish Sauce

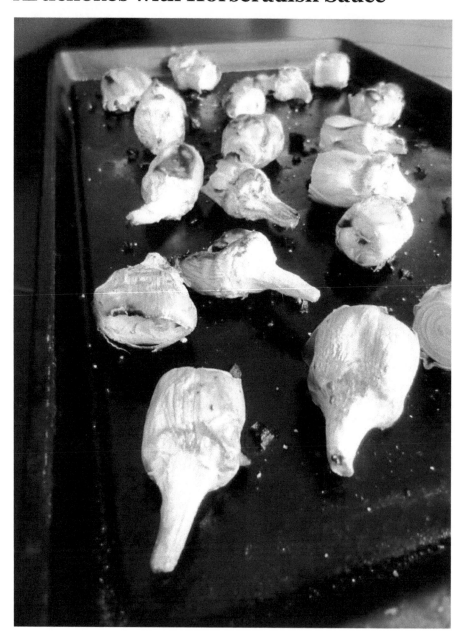

Preparation time: 10 minutes Cooking time: 45 minutes Servings: 2

Ingredients:

1 tablespoon horseradish, prepared

2 tablespoons mayonnaise

A pinch of sea salt

Black pepper to taste

1 teaspoon lemon juice

3 cups artichoke hearts

1 tablespoon lemon juice

Directions:

1.   In a bowl, mix horseradish with mayo, a pinch of sea salt, black pepper and 1 teaspoon lemon juice, whisk well and leave aside for now.

2.   Arrange artichoke hearts on a lined baking sheet, drizzle 2 tablespoons olive oil over them, 1 tablespoon lemon juice and sprinkle a pinch of salt and some black pepper.

3.   Toss to coat well, place in the oven at 425 degrees F and roast for 45 minutes.

4.   Divide artichoke hearts between plates and serve with the horseradish sauce on top.

5.   Enjoy!

Nutritional value/serving: calories 107, fat 5, fiber 3,3, carbs 14,9, protein 1,7

Grilled Artichokes

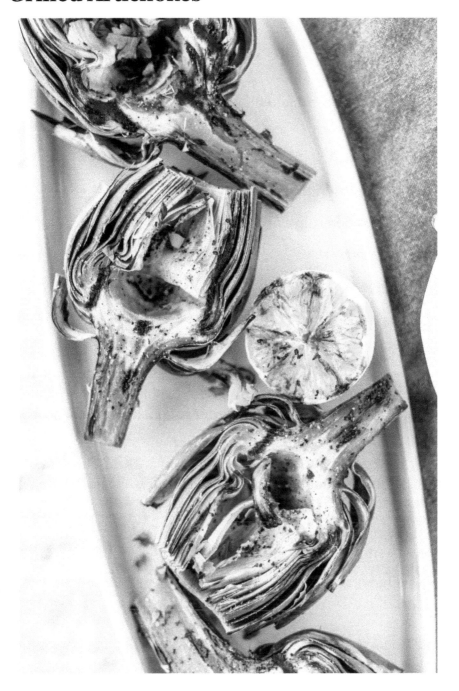

Preparation time: 10 minutes Cooking time: 25 minutes Servings: 4

Ingredients:

2 artichokes, trimmed and halved

Juice of 1 lemon

1   tablespoons lemon zest grated

1 rosemary spring, chopped

2   tablespoons olive oil

A pinch of sea salt

Black pepper to taste

Directions:

1.   Put water in a large saucepan, add a pinch of salt and lemon juice, bring to a boil over medium-high heat, add artichokes, boil for 15 minutes, drain and leave them to cool down.

2.   Drizzle olive oil over them, season with black pepper to taste, sprinkle lemon zest and rosemary, stir well and place them under a preheated grill.

3.   Broil artichokes over medium-high heat for 5 minutes on each side, divide them between plates and serve.

4.   Enjoy!

Nutritional value/serving: calories 98, fat 7,1, fiber 4,4, carbs 8,5, protein 2,7

Artichokes and Tomatoes Dip

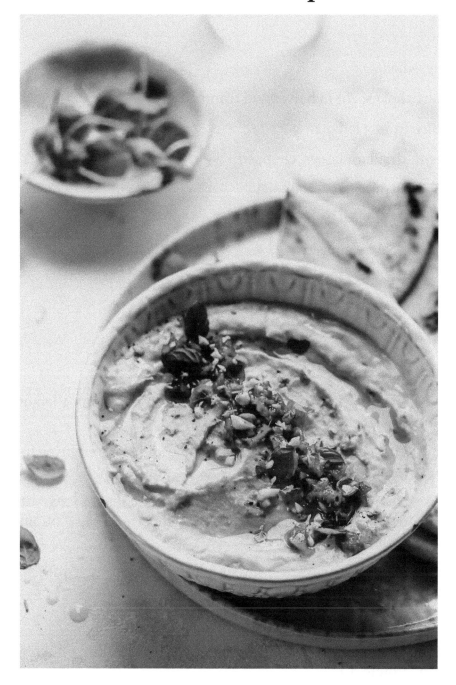

Preparation time: 10 minutes Cooking time: 30 minutes Servings: 4

Ingredients:

2 artichokes, cut in halves and trimmed

Juice from 3 lemons

4 sun-dried tomatoes, chopped

A bunch of parsley, chopped

A bunch of basil, chopped

1 garlic clove, minced

4 tablespoons olive oil

Black pepper to taste

Directions:

1.   In a bowl, mix artichokes with lemon juice from 1 lemon, some black pepper and toss to coat.

2.   Transfer to a large saucepan, add water to cover, bring to a boil over medium-high heat, cook for 30 minutes and drain.

3.   In a food processor, mix the rest of the lemon juice with tomatoes, parsley, basil, garlic, black pepper and olive oil and blend well.

4.   Divide artichokes between plates and top each with the tomatoes dip.

5.   Enjoy!

Nutritional value/serving: calories 193, fat 14,5, fiber 6,1, carbs 16,9, protein 4,1

Carrots and Lime Mix

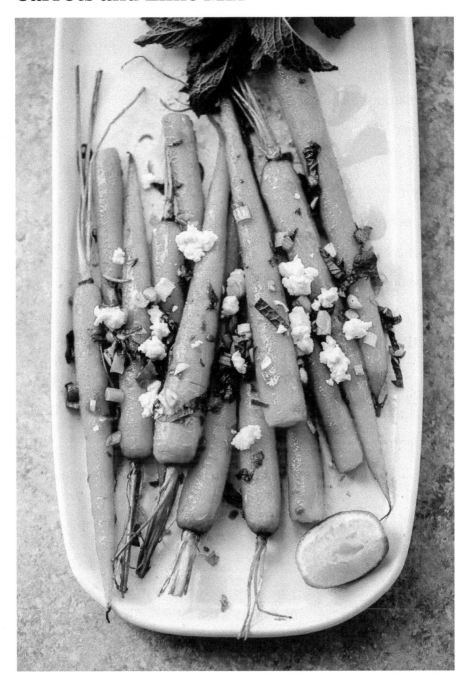

Preparation time: 10 minutes Cooking time: 30 minutes Servings: 6

Ingredients:

1 and ¼ pounds baby carrots

3 tablespoons ghee, melted

8 garlic cloves, minced

A pinch of sea salt

Black pepper to taste

Zest of 2 limes, grated

½ teaspoon chili powder

Directions:

1.   In a bowl, mix baby carrots with ghee, garlic, a pinch of salt, black pepper to taste, chili powder and stir well.

2.   Spread carrots on a lined baking sheet, place in the oven at 400 degrees F and roast for 15 minutes.

3.   Take carrots out of the oven, shake baking sheet, place in the oven again and roast for 15 minutes more.

4.   Divide between plates and serve with lime on top.

5.   Enjoy!

Nutritional value/serving: calories 95, fat 6,6, fiber 2,9, carbs 9,1, protein 0,9

Maple Glazed Carrots

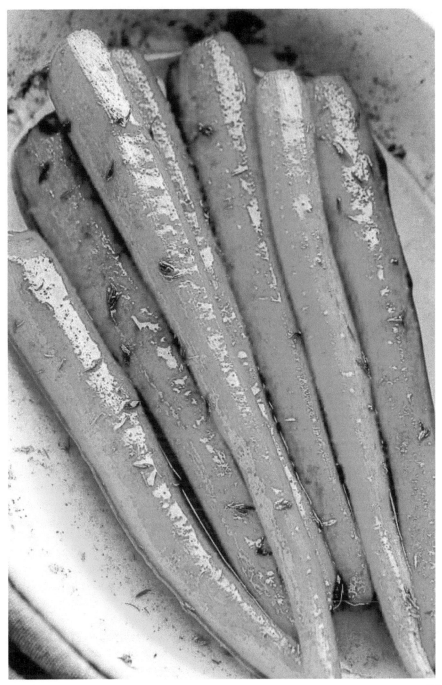

Preparation time: 10 minutes Cooking time: 15 minutes Servings: 4

Ingredients:

1 pound carrots, sliced

1 tablespoon coconut oil

1 tablespoon ghee

½ cup pineapple juice

1 teaspoon ginger, grated

½ tablespoon maple syrup

½ teaspoon nutmeg

1 tablespoon parsley, chopped

Directions:

1.   Heat a pan with the ghee and the oil over medium-high heat, add ginger, stir and cook for 2 minutes.

2.   Add carrots, stir and cook for 5 minutes.

3.   Add pineapple juice, maple syrup and nutmeg, stir and cook for 5 minutes more.

4.   Add parsley, stir, cook for 3 minutes, divide between plates and serve.

5.   Enjoy!

Nutritional value/serving: calories 130, fat 6,8, fiber 3, carbs 17,4, protein 1,1

Purple Carrot Mix

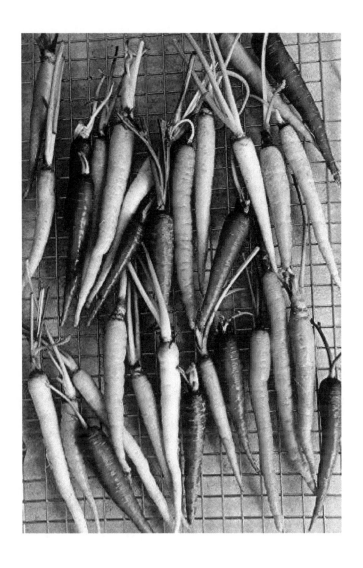

Preparation time: 10 minutes Cooking time: 1 hour Servings: 5

Ingredients:

6 purple carrots, peeled

A drizzle of olive oil

2   tablespoons sesame seeds paste

6 tablespoons water

3   tablespoons lemon juice

1 garlic clove, minced

A pinch of sea salt

Black pepper to taste

White sesame seeds for serving

Directions:

1.   Arrange the purple carrots on a lined baking sheet, sprinkle a pinch of salt, black pepper and a drizzle of oil, place in the oven at 350 degrees F and bake for 1 hour.

2.   Meanwhile, in a food processor, mix sesame seeds paste with water, lemon juice, garlic, a pinch of sea salt and black pepper and pulse well.

3.   Spread over the carrots, toss gently, divide between plates and sprinkle sesame seeds on top.

4.   Enjoy!

Nutritional value/serving: calories 100, fat 4,7, fiber 0,9, carbs 13,6, protein 1,2

Baked Potatoes and "BBQ" Lentils

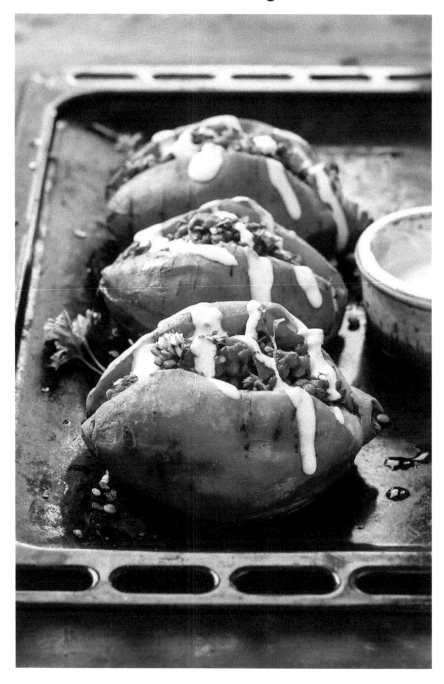

Preparation Time: 5 mins Servings: 4

Ingredients:

2 sliced large baked potatoes

1 c. dry brown lentils

2 tsps. molasses

1 chopped small onion

2 tsps. liquid smoke

3 c. water

½ c. organic ketchup

Directions:

1.   Add water, onion and lentils to the pot

2.   Lock up the lid and cook on HIGH pressure for 10 minutes

3.   Release the pressure naturally

4.   Add ketchup, liquid smoke and molasses to the lentil

5.   Sauté for 5 minutes

6.   Serve over baked potatoes and enjoy!

Nutrition: Calories: 140, Fat:4 g, Carbs:24 g, Protein:5 g, Sugars:606 g, Sodium:18 mg

Superb Lemon Roasted Artichokes

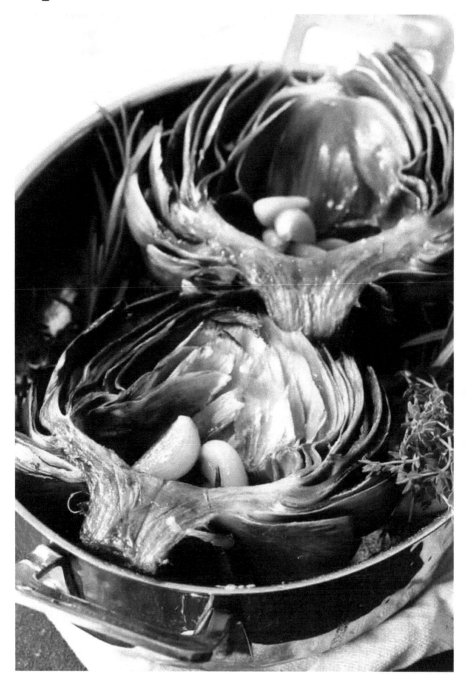

Preparation Time: 10 mins Servings: 2

Ingredients

2 peeled and sliced garlic cloves

3 lemon pieces

Black pepper

2 artichoke pieces

3 tbsps. olive oil

Sea flavored vinegar

Directions:

1. Wash your artichokes well and dip them in water and cut the stem to about ½ inch long

2. Trim the thorny tips and outer leaves and rub the chokes with lemon

3. Poke garlic slivers between the choke leaves and place a trivet basket in the Instant Pot ten add artichokes

4. Lock up the lid and cook on high pressure for 7 minutes

5. Release the pressure naturally over 10 minutes

6. Transfer the artichokes to cutting board and allow them to cool then cut half lengthwise and cut the purple white center

7. Pre-heat your oven to 400 degree Fahrenheit

8. Take a bowl and mix 1 and ½ lemon and olive oil

9. Pour over the choke halves and sprinkle flavored vinegar and pepper

10. Place an iron skillet in your oven and heat it up for 5 minutes

11. Add a few teaspoon of oil and place the marinated artichoke halves in the skillet

12. Brush with lemon and olive oil mixture

13. Cut third lemon in quarter and nestle them between the halves

14. Roast for 20-25 minutes until the chokes are browned

15. Serve and enjoy!

Nutrition: Calories: 263, Fat:16 g, Carbs:8 g, Protein:23 g, Sugars:128 g, Sodium:0.4 mg

Fat Free Apple Cake

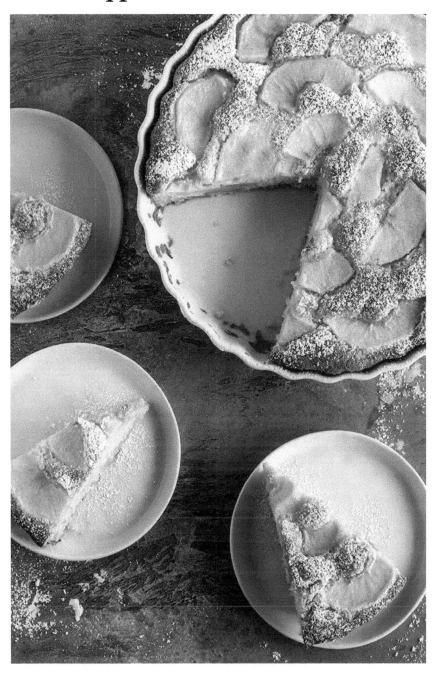

Preparation Time: 20 Minutes Servings: 8

Ingredients:

2   granny smith apples, peeled, cored, and diced

1¾ cups unbleached all-purpose flour

⅔ cup packed light brown sugar

½ cup applesauce

1 tablespoon freshly squeezed lemon juice

1½ teaspoons ground cinnamon

1 teaspoon pure vanilla extract

1 teaspoon baking powder

½ teaspoon baking soda

½ teaspoon salt

¼ teaspoon ground allspice

¼ teaspoon ground nutmeg

⅛ teaspoon ground cloves

Directions:

1.   Lightly oil a baking tray that will fit in the steamer basket of your Instant Pot.

2.   In a bowl, combine the flour, baking powder, baking soda, sugar, cinnamon, allspice, nutmeg, cloves, and salt.

3.   In another bowl combine the applesauce, vanilla, and lemon juice.

4.   Fold in the diced apples.

5.   Stir the wet mixture into the dry mixture slowly until they form a smooth mix.

6.   Pour the batter into your baking tray and put the tray in your steamer basket.

7.   Pour the minimum amount of water into the base of your Instant Pot and lower the steamer basket.

8.   Seal and cook on Steam for 12 minutes.

9.   Release the pressure quickly and set to one side to cool a little.

Pina-Colada Cake

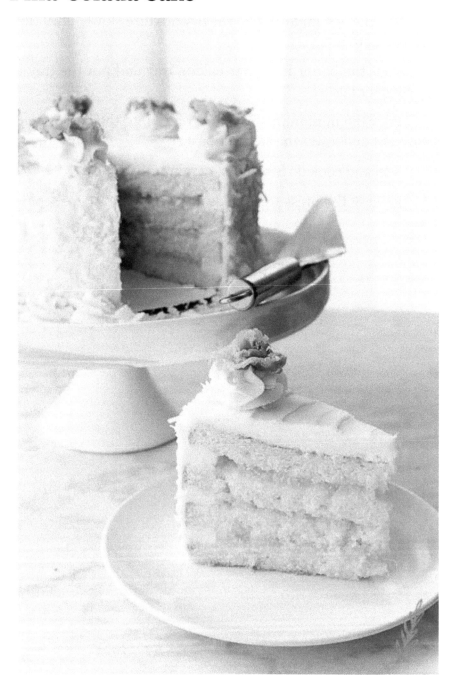

Preparation Time: 20 Minutes Servings: 6

Ingredients:

2 cups unbleached all-purpose flour 1 cup cream of coconut

1 cup confectioners' sugar

¾ cup canned pineapple, well drained, juice reserved

⅓ cup packed light brown sugar or granulated natural sugar

¼ cup unsweetened shredded coconut

3 tablespoons vegan butter, softened, or vegetable oil

1 tablespoon dark rum or 1 teaspoon rum extract

1½ teaspoons baking powder

1 teaspoon apple cider vinegar

½ teaspoon salt

½ teaspoon baking soda

½ teaspoon coconut extract

Directions:

1.   Lightly oil a baking tray that will fit in the steamer basket of your Instant Pot.

2.   In a bowl combine the flour, sugar, shredded coconut, baking soda, baking powder, and salt.

3.   In another bowl combine the cream of coconut, pineapple juice and flesh, rum, vinegar, and coconut extract.

4.   Combine the wet and dry mixes and stir well to ensure they are evenly combined.

5.   Pour the batter into your baking tray and put the tray in your steamer basket.

6.   Pour the minimum amount of water into the base of your Instant Pot and lower the steamer basket.

7.   Seal and cook on Steam for 12 minutes.

8.   Release the pressure quickly and set to one side to cool a little.

9.   When the cake is cool glaze with a light mix of confectioners' sugar and water.

Pumpkin Spice Cake

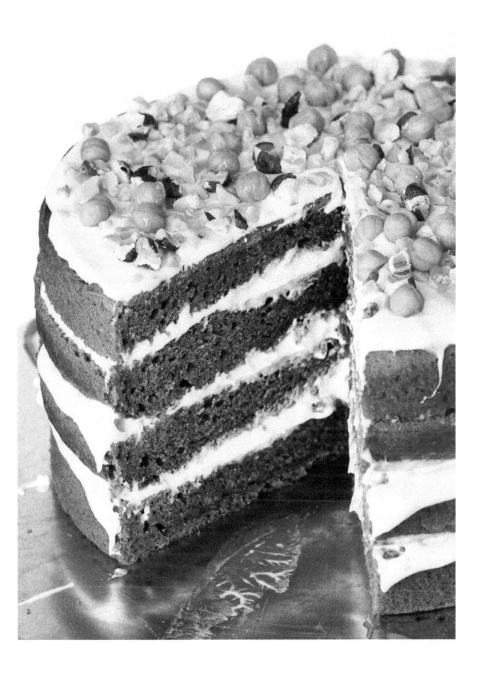

Preparation Time: 28 Minutes Servings: 6

Ingredients:

1¾ cups unbleached all-purpose flour

1 cup canned solid-pack pumpkin

¾ cup packed light brown sugar or granulated natural sugar

½ cup chopped pecans

¼ cup unsweetened almond milk

¼ cup vegetable oil

1½ teaspoons baking powder

1 teaspoon ground cinnamon

1 teaspoon pure vanilla extract

½ teaspoon salt

½ teaspoon ground nutmeg

½ teaspoon ground allspice

¼ teaspoon ground cloves

Directions:

1.   Lightly oil a baking tray that will fit in the steamer basket of your Instant Pot.

2.   In a bowl combine the flour, baking powder, cinnamon, nutmeg, allspice, cloves, sugar, and salt.

3.   In another bowl combine the pumpkin, oil, almond milk, and vanilla.

4.   Mix the wet and dry mixtures together until the mix is evenly smooth.

5.   Fold in the pecans.

6.   Pour the batter into your baking tray and put the tray in your steamer basket.

7.   Pour the minimum amount of water into the base of your Instant Pot and lower the steamer basket.

8.   Seal and cook on Steam for 12 minutes.

9.   Release the pressure quickly and set to one side to cool a little.

Lightning Source UK Ltd.
Milton Keynes UK
UKHW021014030521
383041UK00001B/112

9 781801 458115